KNOW YOUR POISON NO. 4: IV PROPOFOL

An Indian Society of Toxicology Initiative

Dr Vivekanshu Verma
Dr Vijay Vasudev Pillay
Dr Shiv Rattan Kochar
Dr Prateek Rastogi
Dr Karen Harshita

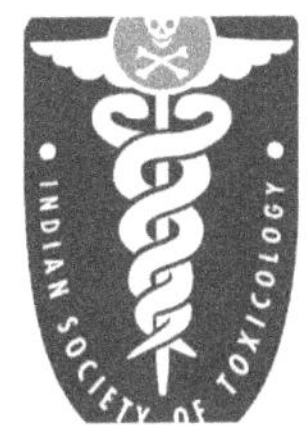

ISBN: 9798711313724

Cover design by: Vishwendra Verma
Library of Indian Society of Toxicology Archive Number: 2018675309
Printed in the Poison Control Centre
Amrita Institute of Medical Science,
Ponekkara, P. O, Kochi, Kerala - 682041.

CONTENTS

KNOW YOUR POISON NO. 4:

IV Propofol: Toxic Riddle for the Toxic Detective

An Indian Society of Toxicology Initiative

For Toxic Detectives, Crime Scene Investigators (CSi), Toxicologists, Police Officers, CID & CBI officers, Lawyers, Judges, Magistrates, Legal counsels, Law Students, Forensic Scientists, Doctors, Toxicology Nurses & Emergency Paramedics

Dr Vivekanshu Verma, MBBS, Postgraduate Diploma in Forensic Medicine & Toxicology, Fellow of Indian Society of Toxicology, Associate Consultant, Emergency & Trauma care, Medanta-The Medicity, Gurugram. Honorary Toxicology Expert, Central Bureau of Investigation

Dr Vijay Vasudev Pillay, MBBS, MD Forensic Medicine & Toxicology, Chief, Poison Control Centre, Professor & Head, Forensic Medicine & Toxicology, Amrita School of Medicine, Amrita Vishwa Vidyapeetham, Cochin, Kerala

Dr Shiv Rattan Kochar, MBBS, MD Forensic Medicine & Toxicology, Senior Professor & Head, Department of Forensic Medicine & Toxicology, Sardar Patel Medical college, Bikaner (Rajasthan)

Dr Prateek Rastogi, MBBS, MD, PGDMLE, PGDCFS, PGCMNCPA, PGCTM, Dip. Cyber Law, FAGE, FAIMER Fellow (MUFILIPE-Manipal), Former President, Indian Society of Toxicology (2018-19), Professor, Department of Forensic Medicine & Toxicology, Kasturba Medical College, Mangalore, Karnataka

Dr Karen Harshita, MD Forensic Medicine & Toxicology, Senior Resident, Department of Forensic Medicine & Toxicology, Chamarajanagar Institute of Medical Sciences, Chamarajanagar, Karnataka

ISBN: 9798711313724

Know your Poison No. 4: IV Propofol: Toxic Riddle for the Toxic Detective

Vivekanshu Verma
Dr Vijay Vasudev Pillay
Dr Shiv Rattan Kochar
Dr Prateek Rastogi
Dr Karen Harshita

An Indian Society of Toxicology Initiative

WHAT'S in Poison's NAME (ETYMOLOGY) OF Propofol: AS YOU LIKE IT!

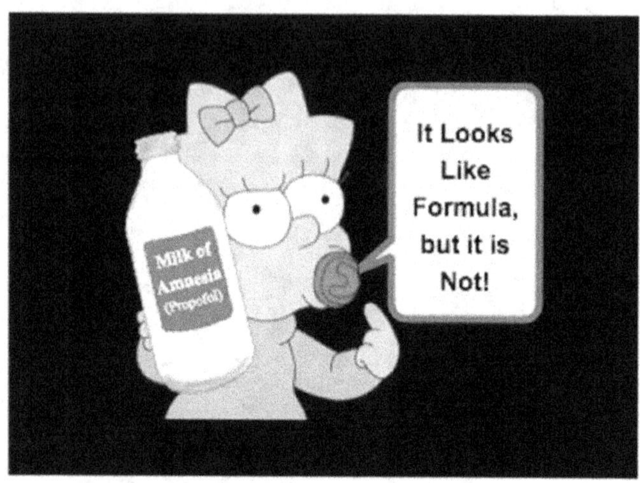

Toximonic of "Falls on All IV = 4" for Easy Recall

Prop-O-fol = pronounced as "Prop 'O' Fall"

- Prop means to keep from falling or slipping by providing a support under or against
- Fall is a 4-letter word, so propofol causes rapid fall in all vitals
- "IV" means 4 as roman number
- IV stands for Intra Venous, as propofol is injected as intravenous anesthetic.

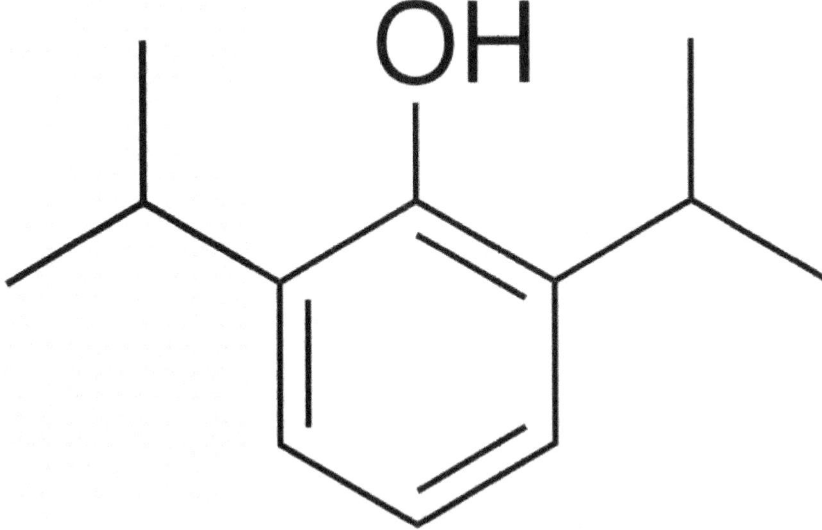

Figure 1. Propofol molecular structure in 2 -D. Image source: Harbin (Wikipedia)

PROP-O-FOL

1) Fall in GCS (coma inducer)- thus the victim is knocked down, can't stand on all 4 limbs
2) Fall in Intracranial pressure (ICP): helpful in Head injury & acute Brain Stroke
3) Fall in Memory: Propofol is known as milk of amnesia by anesthetics
4) Fall in seizure rates recurrence during status epilepticus

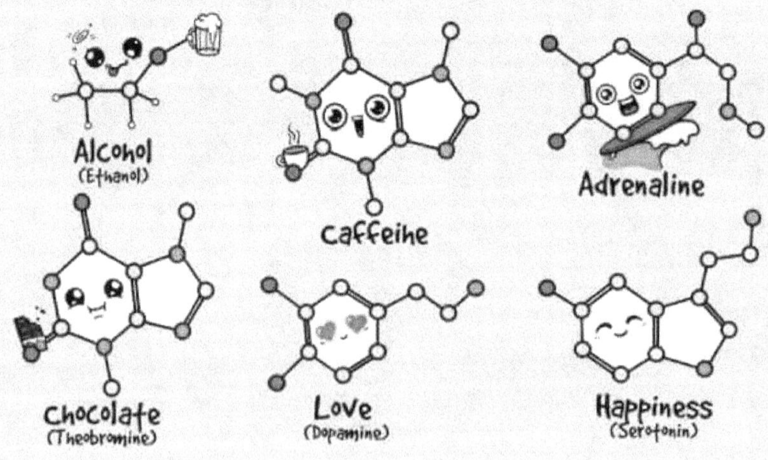

OVERDOSE OF IV-PROPOFOL

causes iatrogenic complications:

- Fall in Breath rate (bradypnea) can cause apnea & decreased response to PaCO2 & PaO2 -> have to provide controlled ventilation if using boluses.
- Fall in Blood Pressure (causes vasodilation and negative inotropy -> hypotension)
- Fall in renal function: decrease renal blood flow and GFR from hypotension
- Fall in muscle power by Rhabdomyolysis due to uncoupling of oxidative phosphorylation in mitochondrial ETC (electronic transport chain)
- Fall in Pulse rate of Heart (bradyarrhythmia)
- Fall in pancreatic function due to excess load of fatty acids in propofol infusion on prolonged use, causing pancreatitis

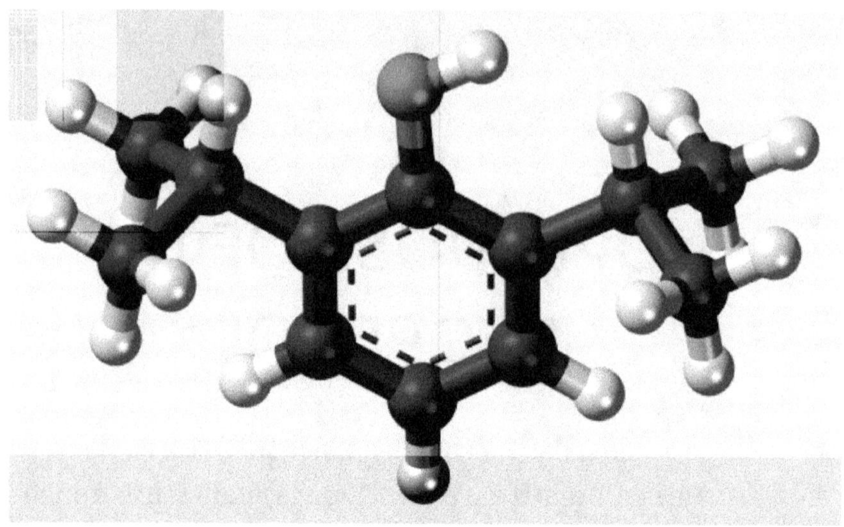

Figure 20. Propofol molecular structure in 3-D Ball & stick model. Image source: Jynto (Wikipedia)

FALL IS FOUR LETTER WORD:

All 4's for easy recall:

4- IV major indications of propofol use in allopathy:

1) Induction + maintenance of General Anaesthesia
2) Procedural Sedation for bronchoscopy, Upper gastrointestinal endoscopy, colonoscopy, sigmoidoscopy (Procedure done in posing on All 4's)
3) Status Epilepticus & Eclampsia, may provide some cerebral protection
4) Status Asthmaticus: bronchodilator properties may be useful in treating bronchospasms

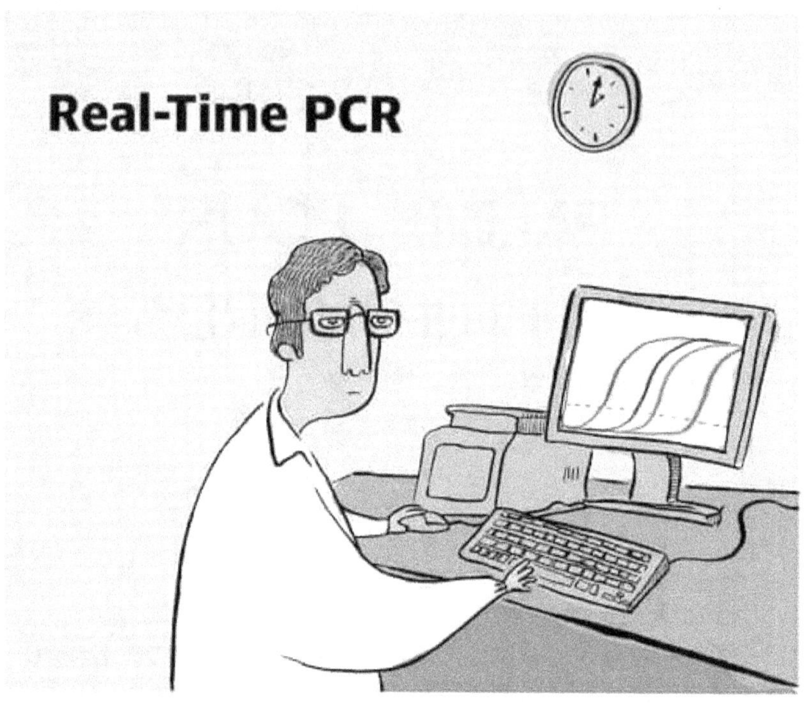
Real-Time PCR

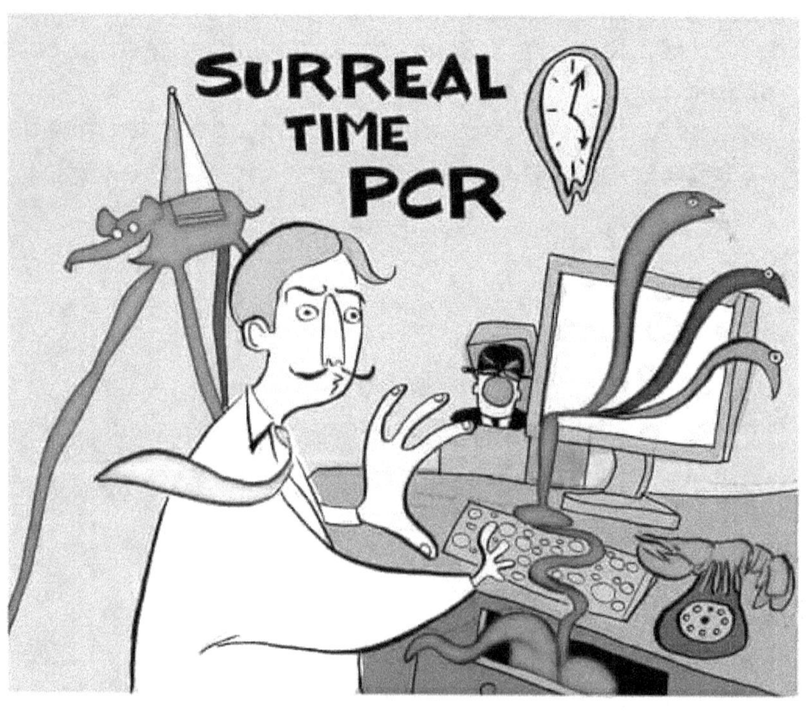
SURREAL
TIME
PCR

4- IV NURSING TIPS:

Do's & Don'ts for propofol injection:

- SHAKE WELL BEFORE USE
- infuse undiluted; if there is a need to dilute prior to administration, use only dextrose 5%.
- Do not dilute to a concentration <2mg/mL
- Do not use if evidence of separation of the emulsion
- must change IV tubing and bottles q12h when running as a continuous infusion
- maintain strict aseptic technique during handling as vehicle can support rapid bacterial growth

IV- 4- EMERGENCY TIPS:

Do's & Don'ts for propofol usage:
All 4's & P's for easy recall

- P-Prefer 4 hour NPO (Nil Per Mouth) before P-Procedural sedation
- P-Pressure over cricoid during rapid sequence intubation to P-Prevent aspiration
- P-Proton Pump Inhibitors – P-Pantoprazole is helpful as Prophylaxis for acid reflux

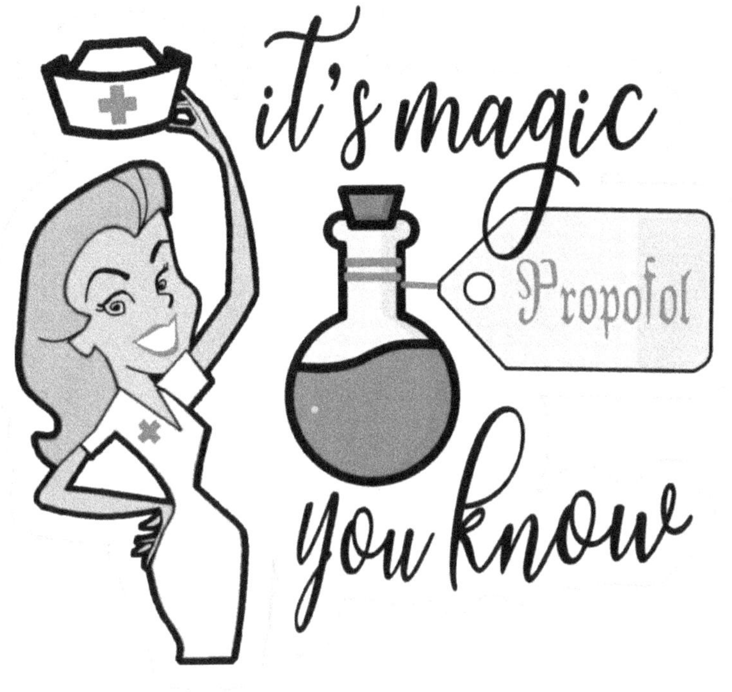

4- MAJOR USES OF IV PROPOFOL

*for non- therapeutic purposes
(off-label use):*

1) Recreational misuse among Operation theatre related anesthetics, staff & paramedics
2) Legal execution for causing sudden death during capital punishment in west
3) Drug abuse for refractory insomnia (As the case of Michael Jackson Popstar's death)
4) Veterinary use for chemically restraining the violent mad wild animals: elephants

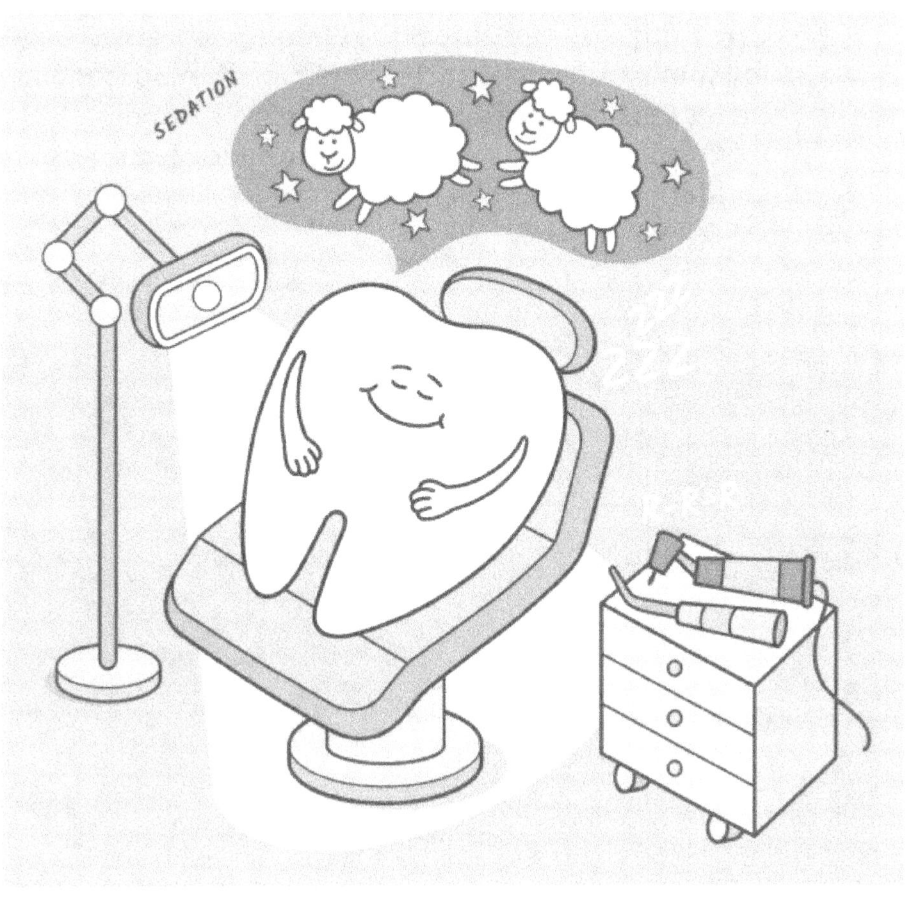

IV- 4- UNIQUE FACTS OF PROPOFOL:

- Its not listed as narcotic, not covered under Narcotic Drugs & Psychotropic Substances Act
- It can be given by Registered Nurses in absence of doctors, to intubated, ventilated patients

- Unwillingness of insurers to reimburse anesthesia care for some procedures such as diagnostic endoscopy has increased the use of nurse-administered propofol.
- Its Continuous infusion is not recommended for use in children < 18 years of age.

ALL IV- 4'S FOR EASY RECALL FOR DOSES OF PROPOFOL: -

- Propofol induction Bolus –2mg/kg (half of four) approx.. 40mg q10sec
- Onset of action: within 40 seconds of IV injection
- Maintenance dose of propofol infusion: 4 – 12mcg/kg/min
- Children: induction dose: increase dose by 40% -> maintenance: increase by 40%
- Plasma concentrations: sedation <2 mcg/mL, hypnosis: 2 – 6 mcg/mL (=4mcg/mL approx..)
- Maintenance of ICU sedation: <0.4mg/kg/hour, increased by increments of 0.4mg/kg/h over q5min until desired level of sedation is achieved.

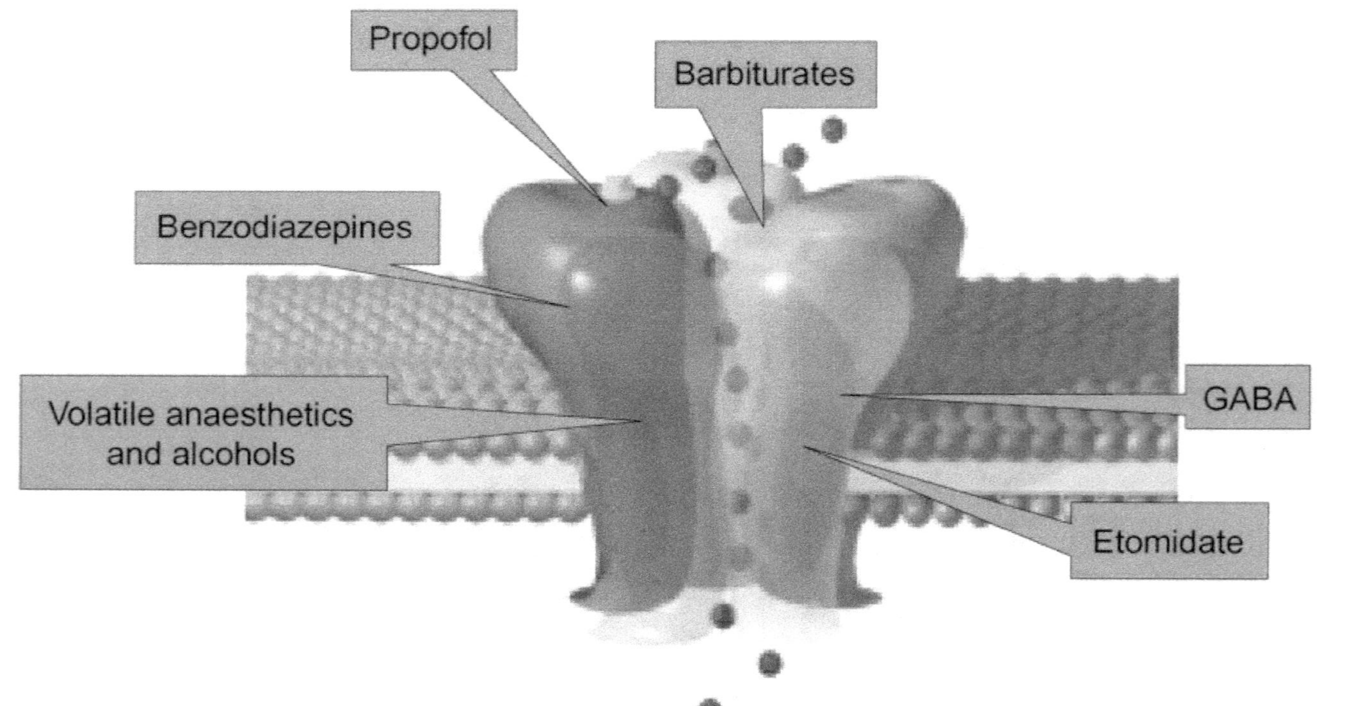

Cartoon representation of the g-aminobutyric acid (GABA)-A receptor sitting in a cell membrane, indicating some of the drug binding sites. The spots represent chloride ions flowing through the channel. Reprinted from Drug Discovery Today, Vol. 8, Whiting PJ. GABA-A receptor subtypes in the brain: a paradigm for CNS drug discovery? p. 448, 2003, with permission from Elsevier.

MECHANISM OF ACTION

*NMDA & GABA: Both 4 -letter
word for IV propofol:*

Propofol works via activation of central GABA pathways and inhibition of NMDA (N-Methyl-DL-aspartic-acid) pathways.

- P-Positive modulation of GABA: 4 letter acronyms for Gamma Amino Butyric Acid, an inhibitory neurotransmitter acting on the cerebrospinal locations for rapid sedation

IV- 4 ADVANTAGES OF PROPOFOL: ALL 4'S FOR EASY RECALL:

1) Rapid onset (within 40 seconds)
2) Rapid offset (within 4 minutes)
3) Lipid soluble, so rapidly enters, into cerebral circulation, crossing blood brain barriers easily.
4) Propofol is often used instead of sodium thiopental for starting anesthesia because recovery from propofol is more rapid and "clear" without any memory of the surgery

IV- 4 CO-CONSTITUENTS OF PROPOFOL

for concern on administration:

1)   Purified Egg phosphatide: causes anaphylaxis reaction in patients with egg allergy. Egg white gives white milky colour to the bottle of propofol. Lecithin from egg yolk is added for emulsifying to dissolve the oil-in-water emulsion

2)   Sulfite preservative may cause drug allergy in some, but its not associated to sulfa medications. Sulfites & sulfa medications are chemically unrelated, but they can both cause allergic reactions.

3)   Soybean oil: causes anaphylaxis reaction in patients with soyabean allergy

4)   Sodium Hydroxide (NaOH): corrosive base added as preservative, causes local burning painful sensation at site of infusion

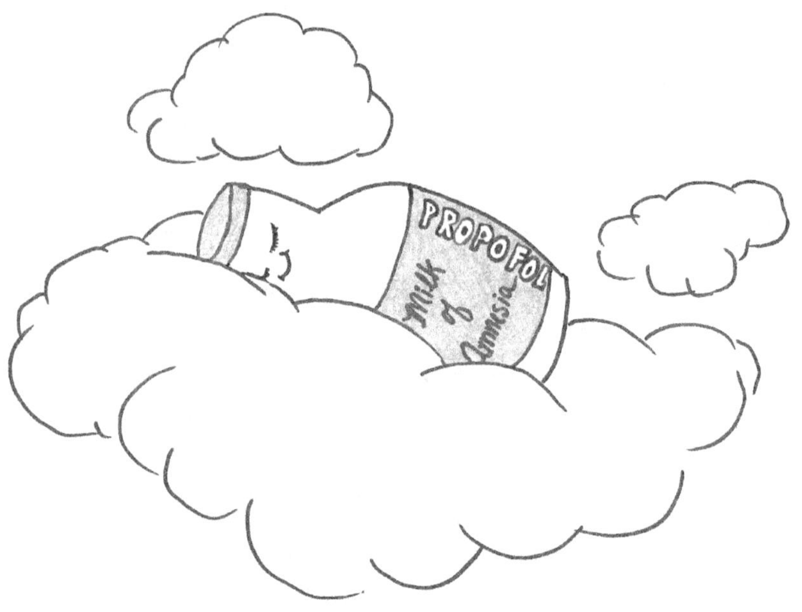
PROPOFOL
milk of amnesia

P-PROPOFOL IS SAFE TO USE IN ALL P'S:

Toximonic of all P's for easy recall:

1) P-Pregnancy – it is helpful in induction during caesarean delivery
2) P-Preeclampsia included status epilepticus
3) P-Pediatrics- its safe to use in kids for daycare surgeries
4) P-Porphyria- Propofol is safe to use in patients suffering from Porphyria

4 TARGET ORGANS

in Propofol toxicity:

1) Cardiovascular:
- Hypotension
- Dysrhythmias (ex, Bradycardia, Wide QRS, Brugada-like ECG, VTach, PEA, asystole)
- Myocardial Failure

2) Metabolic (uncoupling oxidative phosphorylation in mito-chondria)
- Hyperthermia
- Metabolic Acidosis

3) Renal and Musculoskeletal:
- Rhabdomyolysis
- Acute Renal Failure

4) Hepatic:
- Hepatomegaly and Transaminitis
- Hypertriglyceridemia and Lipdemia

TOXICITY OF IV-PROPOFOL IN UNCONSCIOUS VICTIMS:

- ABG: Hypoxia, metabolic acidosis & rise in lactates
- ECG- ST depression, dysrhythmia
- USG: 2d Echo: severe LV dysfunction due to toxic cardiomyopathy
- Urine discoloration: Green / Brown due to rhabdomyolysis

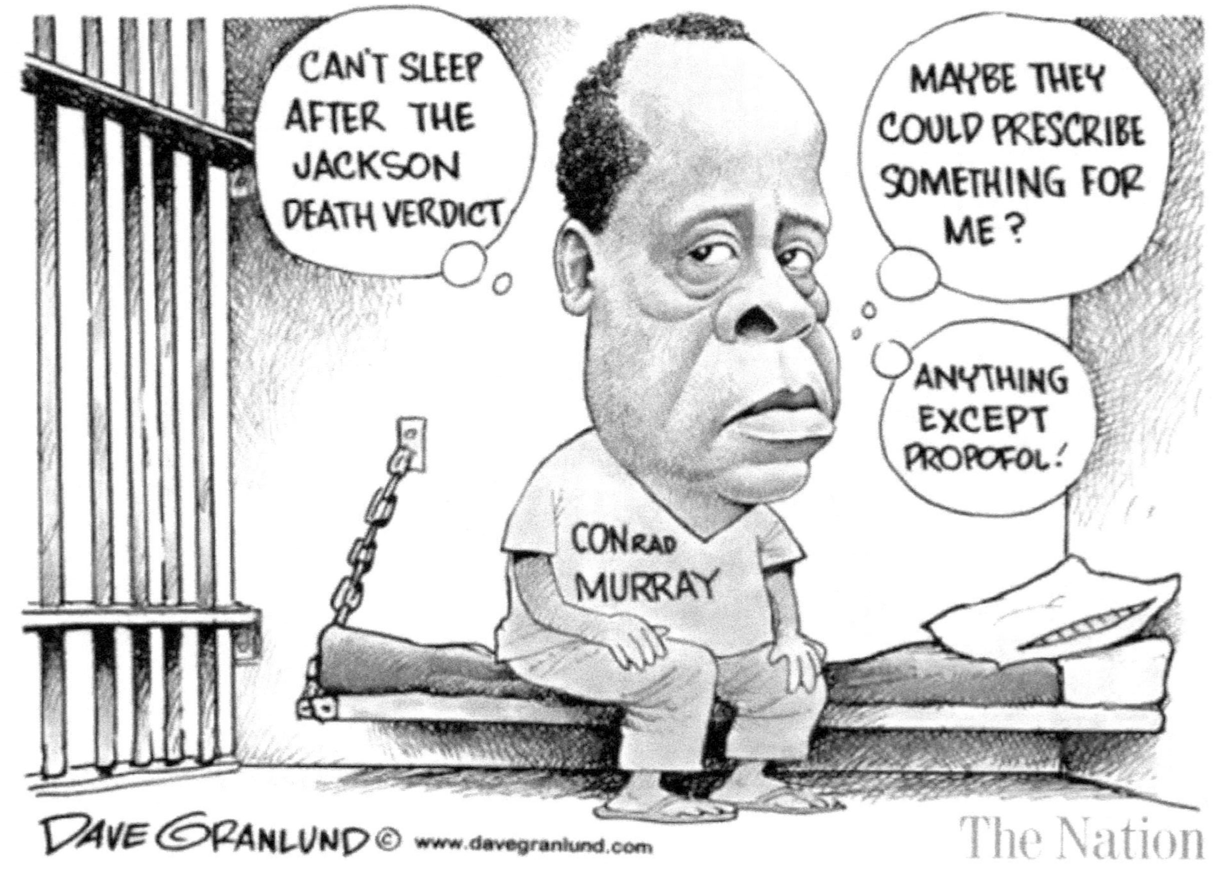
CAN'T SLEEP AFTER THE JACKSON DEATH VERDICT
MAYBE THEY COULD PRESCRIBE SOMETHING FOR ME?
ANYTHING EXCEPT PROPOFOL!
CONRAD MURRAY
DAVE GRANLUND © www.davegranlund.com
The Nation

POPSTAR MICHAEL JACKSON'S DEATH

By iatrogenic propofol overdose

After 22 days of testimony and less than two days of deliberation, a jury found Michael Jacksons personal doctor, Conrad Murray, guilty of involuntary manslaughter, nearly two and a half years after the singers drug-related death. Prosecutors argued that Murray was grossly negligent in administering an anaesthetic called propofol to help Jackson sleep.

A fatal dose of the powerful drug, normally used for surgery, was ruled to be the main cause of the King of Pops death at age 50.
The defence argued that Jackson delivered the fatal dose himself.
He is a primary care physician, not an anaesthesiologist, and thus should not have been administering propofol at all.
He also kept no records of administering the drug, did not use proper monitoring equipment, failed to immediately call 911 after discovering the singer unconscious, and didn't alert paramedics on the scene about Jacksons propofol use.

During the four-week case, prosecutors portrayed Murray as a deceptive and incompetent doctor who abandoned his medical judgment by administering a surgical drug to Jackson in order to help him sleep.

The prosecution brought in key witnesses who testified to many egregious medical missteps, which experts said directly led to Jacksons death.

(Opinion of NY Times, LA Times, Telegraph...) The Week Link: https://nation.com.pk/10-Nov-2011/the-conrad-murray-verdict-5-takeaways
:

PRIS: IV

- 4's for easy recall with Propofol Infusion Syndrome
(PRIS): PRIS is the 4-letter word:-
- Doses of >4mg/kg/hr for >48 hours associated with-> propofol infusion syndrome
- Blood levels of triglycerides 400 mg/dL or more during fatty emulsion of propofol infused for long time, due to inhibition of fatty acid oxidation

PRIS RELATED EMERGENCIES:

1)   Severe metabolic acidosis due to renal shutdown & elevated lactates because of end organ tissue hypoxia
2)   Bradycardia & arrhythmia (ex, Bradycardia, Wide QRS, Brugada-like ECG, VTach, PEA, asystole)
3)   multiorgan dysfunction (MODS) & failure
4)   treatment resistant cardiac arrest (described mainly in children)

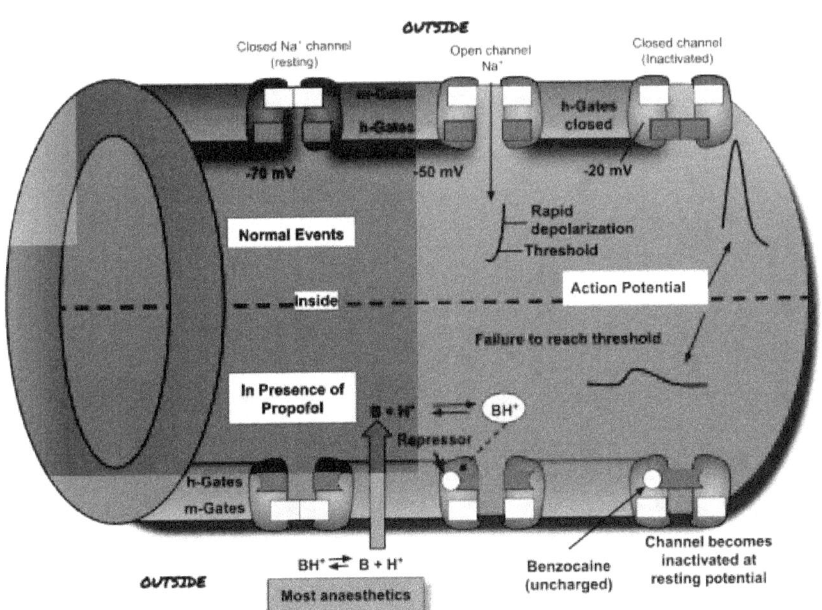

Figure 3. Propofol effect on the mind body

Most local anesthetics are weak bases (B) B + H+ $\rightleftharpoons$ BH+ (protonated form). The relative proportion of the two forms is given by log(BH/B) + B = pKA – pH (e.g. 8.4 – 7.4 = 1). Thus the ionized molecules predominate.

https://www.lhsc.on.ca/critical-care-trauma-centre/propofol-diprivan

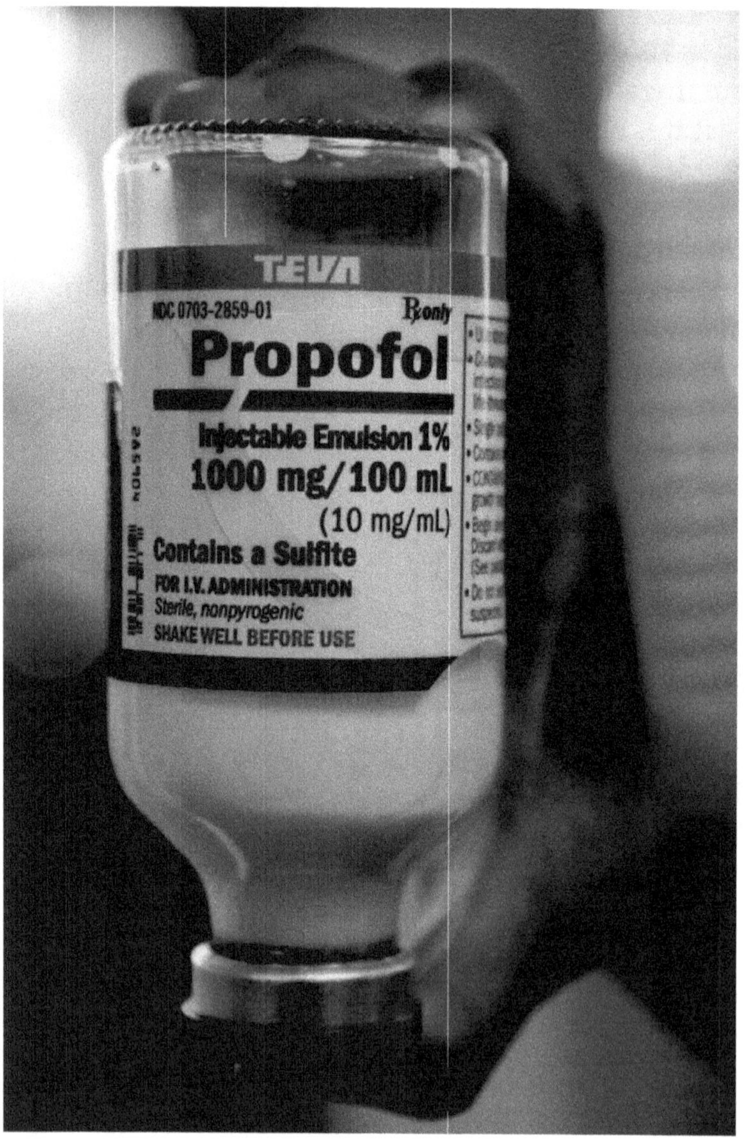

IS PROPOFOL A NARCOTIC?

Propofol is not scheduled under the Controlled Substances Act (CSA).

IS IT NORMAL TO WAKE UP DURING A COLONOSCOPY?

Actually, it shouldn't. Prior to the procedure, patients are given a combination of a narcotic and sedative called "conscious sedation." About 95 percent of patients sleep through the entire procedure and wake up with no memory of the experience.

WHY DOES PROPOFOL BURN SO BAD WHEN INJECTED?

The main disadvantage of propofol is that it often causes people severe pain. This is because propofol is usually injected into a hand vein and can cause skin irritation. This can make the anaesthesia experience unpleasant

DO YOU FEEL PAIN UNDER PROPOFOL?

Propofol has been widely used in clinical practice. However, pain after injection is one of the most common side effects of this intravenous anesthetic. It has been reported that propofol injection pain (PIP) occurred in 60% of untreated patients.

IS PROPOFOL MADE FROM EGGS?

The propofol is mixed in a liquid containing soybean oil and a substance called egg lecithin. Lecithin is a fatty substance found in some plant and animal tissues. Patients who are allergic to foods, including soy and egg, are allergic to proteins in the foods and are not allergic to the oils or fats in the foods.

IS THERE AN ANTIDOTE FOR PROPOFOL?

Unlike other sedation agents (e.g., midazolam, morphine), there is no reversal agent for propofol. Adverse effects must be treated until the drug is metabolized.

CAN NURSES GIVE PROPOFOL IV PUSH?

Administration of IV Anesthetic Agents – Exception.

Registered Nurses, who are competent in the procedure through education and experience, may administer Propofol to intubated, ventilated patients in a critical care setting based on an appropriate medical order.

Unwillingness of insurers to reimburse anesthesia care for some procedures such as diagnostic endoscopy has increased the use of nurse-administered propofol.

INCIDENCE OF PRIS:

"Propofol Infusion Syndrome":

Very rare, but deadly complication coincident with Propofol administration.

True incidence is unknown

May be an extreme manifestation of a more common and initially reversible physiologic state. [Diedrich, 2011]

Causation or mechanism has, as yet, not been determined.

4-IV RISK FACTORS OF PRIS

Through evaluation of the case reports and case series, there appears to be several trends for Risk Factors (although, there are also outliers).

- Dose of Propofol >4 mg/kg/hr
- Duration of Propofol 48 hours or greater
- Patients with Inborn Errors of Metabolism
- Concomitant infusion of Vasopressors
- Concomitant use of Steroids
- Patients with "Critical Illness"
- "Younger" Age – although death seemed to more likely occur in patients >18 years of age.

PRIS: TREATMENT

- There is no specific therapy for Propofol Infusion Syndrome.
o Awareness of it and attempting to prevent it is best option.
o Some recommend monitoring serum lactate levels… but, this obviously is not a diagnostic test.
o Maintaining an adequate carbohydrate load to prevent the increase in fatty acids, hopefully reducing risk.
- Propofol Infusion Syndrome is a diagnosis of exclusion!
o The critically ill patient has many reasons to develop the same clinical features.
o Treat all potential etiologies aggressively (ex, sepsis).
- Supportive Care:
o Stop the propofol once suspicious for this.
o Improve gas exchange
o Cardiac pacing if bradycardic
o Consider glucagon and phosphodiesterase inhibitors
o Hemodialysis
o ECMO (Extra Corporeal Membrane Oxygenation)

MORAL OF THE MORSEL

- Match your Patients and the Sedatives.

As best you are able, consider which medication is right for each specific patient. There is no one perfect medication for everyone.

- Propofol is Powerful. And with great power, comes great responsibility. Use this tool wisely.

- Don't discount your colleagues' experience. While we may have not encountered Propofol Infusion Syndrome in the ED, the PICU's experience may be different.

- Don't throw the Propofol out with the Bathwater.

Over short durations, using appropriate dosages, and in the right patients, the risk of Propofol Infusion Syndrome is likely lower than the risk of the child dislodging the ETT you just placed.

Evaluate your risk assessment scales wisely.

ADVERSE EFFECTS:

Common side effects of propofol include an irregular heart rate, low blood pressure, a burning sensation at the site of injection and the cessation of breathing.

MILK OF AMNESIA

It has been referred to as milk of amnesia (a play on "milk of magnesia"), because of the milk-like appearance of the intravenous preparation, and because of its tendency to suppress memory recall.

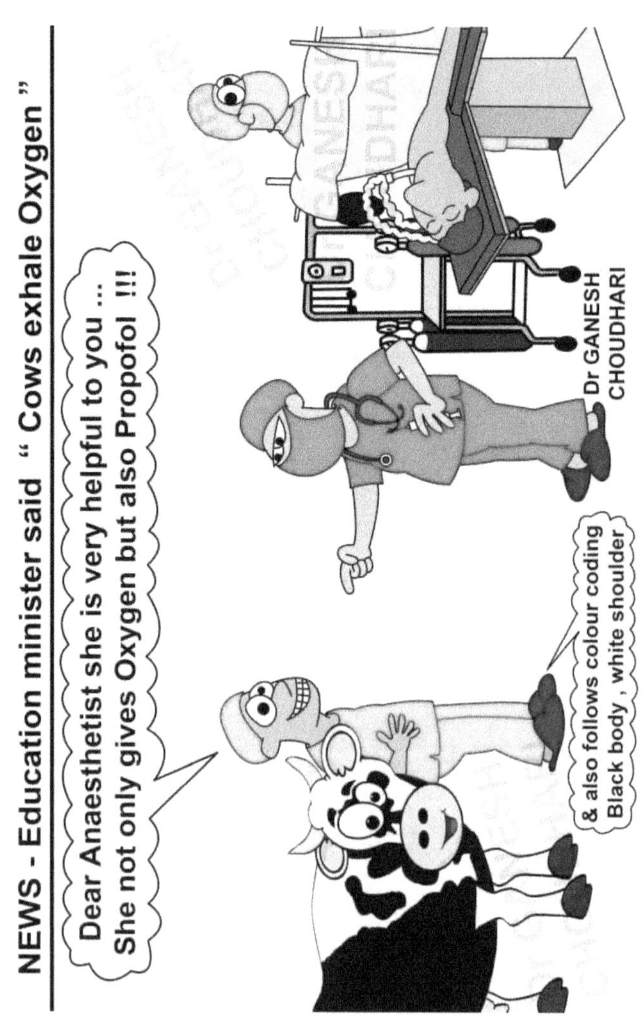

Toximonic of "Falls on All IV 4" for Easy Recall
Prop-O-fol, pronounced as "Prop 'O' Fall"
Prop means to keep from falling or slipping by providing a support under or against
Fall is a 4-letter word, so propofol causes rapid fall in all vitals
"IV" means 4 as roman number
IV stands for Intra Venous, as propofol is injected as intravenous anesthetic

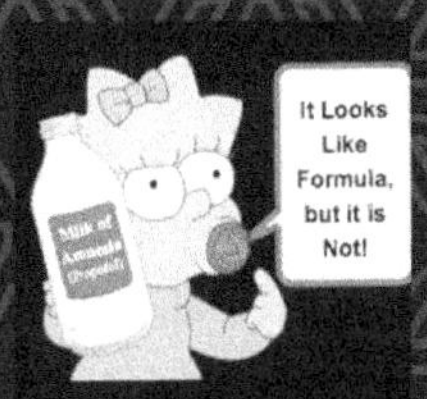

©2021 Indian Society of Toxicology
Poison Control Centre
Amrita Institute of Medical Science, Ponekkara, P. O, Kochi, Kerala - 682041
ISBN: 9798711313724

Vivekanshu Verma
Dr Vijay Vasudev Pillay
Dr Shiv Rattan Kochar
Dr Prateek Rastogi
Dr Karen Harshita

VIAL POETRY

Take a vial its brown or not

Except for Propofol,

Crack it open, leave no drop

Inject a full syringe.

But did you read the BP name

The tiny print and all?

Before you made the patient lame

Embarrassed face; jaws fall.

May I suggest another scheme

To stop this awful fate?

Like Dulux colour coded charts,

Applicate, coordinate.

Make no mistake, a coloured vial

May hide contents therein,

But if you know that blue means slow

And green is paralysing,

Then reds for pain, and you may gain

No room for compromising.

For sceptics and the colour blind

Who have no hope at all,

Then read the damned thing properly

Or you'll go to the wall.

Take a vial, its brown or not

Except for Propofol.

*(Contributed by Dr D. GRAHAM,
Killingbeck Hospital, Leeds LS14 6UQ)*

9 798711 313724